3/18   - 3

HARRIET GRIFFEY

Sit Strong

EVERYDAY EXERCISES TO STRETCH AND STRENGTHEN YOUR POSTURE

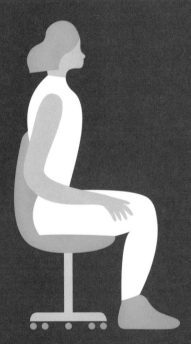

hardie grant books

One.

Two.

Three.

One.

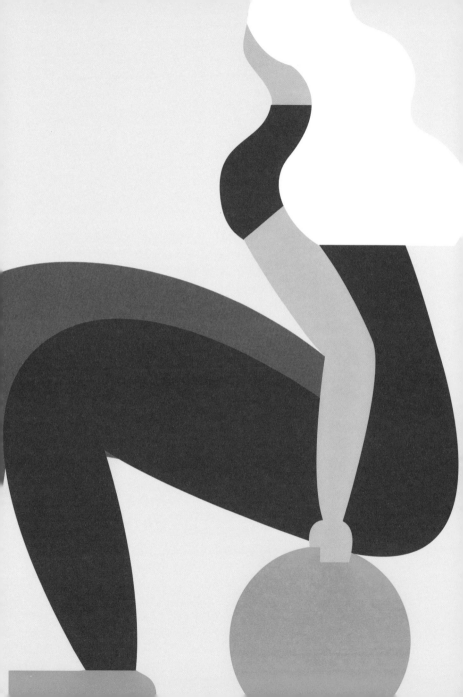

WHY
IT
MATTERS

Our bodies are built for movement. The muscles, ligaments and tendons that support our bones are geared to support an active lifestyle, which should, in turn, keep muscles strong. Without strong muscles the tendons (that connect muscles to bones) or the ligaments (that connect bones to bones) have to take up the slack. However, being fibrous and less flexible, tendons and ligaments can't do the job for which muscles were designed. When muscles are weak, ligaments and tendons take the strain, and this lack of support can put joints at risk. Then, when weak muscles go into spasm, to protect joints from damage, this can result in acute pain. Without proper attention this can easily become a chronic problem. Prevention is always better than cure, especially as ligament strain or tendonitis both take a long time to recover.

HOW BAD IS IT?

It's not just musculoskeletal pain that can result from our sedentary lifestyles. In 2017, the British Heart Foundation (BHF) reported that more than 20 million people in the UK were physically inactive. Their analysis suggested that, on average, British men spent a fifth of their lifetime sitting, which was equivalent to 78 days a year, while for women it was 74 days a year. The report defined 'inactive' as not achieving the minimum government guidelines of

150 minutes of moderate physical activity a week, plus strength-building activities on two days a week. The BHF warned that the risks of this shortfall was an increase in cases of heart disease, which would cost the UK's National Health Service (NHS) around £1.2 billion each year. Physical inactivity, the BHF warned, contributes to more than 5 million deaths worldwide, making it one of the top ten causes of death.

Research shows that a sedentary life is bad for our general health. In addition to increasing the possibility of chronic and debilitating musculoskeletal problems, a stiff achy back, headaches and poor digestion, excessive sitting has been linked to being overweight or obese, to type 2 diabetes, to some types of cancer and even premature death. The good news is that, with a little thought and exercise, there is a huge amount we can do to counteract the effects of sitting and improve our health and wellbeing.

IT'S NEVER TOO LATE

While we're young, being active is relatively easy. As we age and stiffen, it's even more important to keep moving and avoid the worst effects of our sedentary lives – and it's never too late to make a start. Age-related loss of muscle mass begins to occur after the age of 30. We can lose between 2–5 per cent of muscle mass per decade, and this accelerates after the age of 70. This not only weakens us, but makes us more prone to aches, pains and injuries as we age. The technical term for this loss of muscle mass is *sarcopenia* and the more sitting around we do, the worse it gets.

However, it's never too late to make a difference. The great thing about muscles is that they are designed to respond to exercise and it's possible to strengthen and improve muscle tone and mass, whatever your age. It doesn't happen as quickly as when you were in your twenties but it does happen, and both weight-bearing and resistance exercising will make a significant difference over time. So, even if you've done little or no exercise to support your health and fitness for, say, 20 years, your muscle tone can *always* be improved.

In fact, recent research in 2017 from the Mayo Clinic in Rochester, USA, demonstrated unexpectedly good reasons as to why we should exercise when we are older. It seems that the decline associated with ageing at a cellular level in our muscles could be 'corrected' with exercise, especially if that exercise was in intense bursts, according to Dr Sreekumaran Nair, lead author and professor of medicine at the clinic. In fact, in some ways, older people's muscle cells responded more robustly to intense exercise than those of the young, suggesting that it is never too late to benefit from exercise.

Check in with your doctor, a physiotherapist or physical health advisor if you need reassurance, however the gentle exercises in this book, repeated regularly, can form a very positive antidote to sitting.

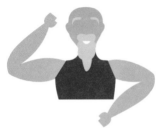

MOVE

Although you may sit for long hours – at work, driving, reading or watching the television – it's important to alternate these periods with those of activity, and consciously factor them into your day to ensure you move enough. This could include walking or cycling to work, getting off the bus a stop or two early, parking as far as you feasibly can from your destination, using the stairs when you can, deliberately getting up from your seat and flexing your body every 30 minutes ... all of which will contribute to keeping you moving. Your waistline will thank you for it, too, and maintaining an optimum weight will also protect your joints from long-term damage.

STRETCH

When we sit slumped for long periods, with shoulders rounded and rotated forwards, we end up with weak muscles in our upper back and neck, and with tight muscles in our shoulders and chest, which puts us at risk of aches and pains. Over time, the lack of movement and the muscular tension caused by the holding patterns we adopt in order to sit for long hours, causes postural problems and pain. Regular, gentle stretching of muscles, tendons and ligaments keeps them supple: set an alarm to go off every 30 minutes, as a reminder to get up from your chair to move and stretch.

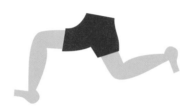

STRENGTHEN

Keeping muscles strong is essential to maintaining good posture and will help, too, to protect you from muscle-ligament- and tendon-strain. Tendons and ligaments compensate for weak muscles, doing a job for which they aren't designed, and this can lead to problems with repetitive strain injuries (RSI). Tendonitis of the elbow, or 'tennis elbow', for example, can be the result of poor muscle tone in the arms and overuse of a computer mouse. Keeping the muscles in your upper back, arms, and even your abdominal core, strong, will help to protect your whole body from long hours spent sitting.

The Benefits of
Being a Fidget-Bottom

In 2016, the *American Journal of Preventive Medicine* published a report from the Department of Epidemiology and Public Health at University College London in which the researchers had looked at whether the more you fidgeted, the better it might be for your health. Researchers used data from the UK Women's Cohort Study, which looked at average sitting time, overall fidgeting (irrespective of posture) and a range of other factors that included physical activity, diet, smoking, and alcohol consumption. Participants were studied over a period of 12 years. The good news is that the report concluded that fidgeting may reduce the risk of all-cause mortality associated with excessive sitting!

CHECK YOUR POSTURE!

Sitting for long periods is surprisingly tiring and, as we tire, so do our muscles, which makes our posture slump further. Sitting slumped becomes a habit and this further aggravates poor posture. Focusing on improving posture includes making sure that where you sit and work is ergonomically suitable. Many of the exercises outlined here will help strengthen your posture generally, whether your are sitting, standing or walking, but here's a checklist to make sure you know how to protect your body while sitting and working at a desk – this is particularly relevant when working on a computer or laptop.

- ✷   Make sure your head is aligned above your shoulders, with your chin tucked in.

- ✷   Sit upright and back into the seat of your chair, using the chair's lumbar support, or a small cushion, to help support your lower back and keep your posture upright.

- ✷   Your thighs should be at a right angle to your hips and your feet should be flat on the floor. If you need to use a low footstool to maintain this position comfortably, do. It will pay dividends in terms of keeping your sitting posture strong.

- ✷   Your computer screen should be directly in front of your eyes, so you don't have to look up or down. If you use a laptop at your workstation, consider raising it up to eye level and using a separate keyboard.

- ✷   Shoulders should be relaxed, neither raised nor hunched forward, with your upper arms and elbows close to your body.

❋ Your keyboard should be at elbow height when you are seated, so your forearms are at a right angle to your upper arm – this also helps to keep shoulders relaxed and lowered.

❋ When typing, your wrists should be straight, parallel to the floor. If you work habitually on a laptop, consider using a separate mouse.

❋ Take regular breaks every 30 minutes, at least, to walk around and run through some stretches.

❋ In addition, it's becoming more of a trend to stand and work at a workstation, in an attempt to counteract the effects of long hours spent sitting. This may be worth considering if you work consistently at a computer, helping to protect your physical health.

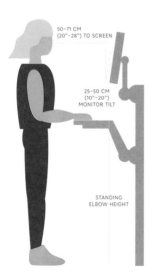

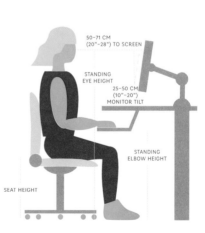

Exercise ball/stability ball/pilates ball/posture ball ... replacing your desk chair with one of these can go a long way to alleviating some of the problems that arise from sitting. This is because an exercise ball is relatively unstable and constantly shifts a little under your weight, demanding that your core muscles work to keep you upright. These micro-adjustments that your body has to continually make, keeps your muscular activity 'switched on', even in your legs, and this helps to strengthen your muscles, compensating a little for long hours spent sitting.

VARIFOCAL GLASSES

Be aware that if you wear varifocal glasses at the computer for long periods of time, this can cause strain on the neck. Viewing the computer screen through the bottom of the lens makes you tilt your head and push your chin forward and this will compress the back of your neck. over time, this position can cause muscle fatigue, tightness and pain. You can help avoid this by placing the computer screen at a lower level but it's better to use single lens glasses for extensive computer use. Ask your optician for advice about what glasses would suit you best for 'computer use' to avoid neck strain. (See also page 27.)

Using This Book

This book shows you what you can do to strengthen your body and improve flexibility, to specifically counteract the risk to health of long hours spent sitting. Divided into six main sections – head and neck; shoulders and upper back; arms; fingers, hands and wrists; lower back and bottom; and legs – it will lead you through a simple series of routine exercises, designed to target areas that can be badly affected. There are specific exercises to stretch and strengthen, to release the muscle tension that aggravates problems, and to support posture.

Bear in mind that although the exercises are divided into six sections, there is inevitably a link between them, which is why there is also a section on how to put it all together for the benefit of the whole body.

Simple to do, and easy to incorporate into your day, devising your personal exercise plan takes just minutes and pays dividends. Start today and feel better immediately.

Two.

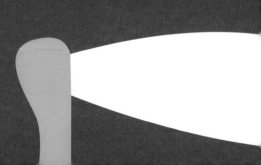

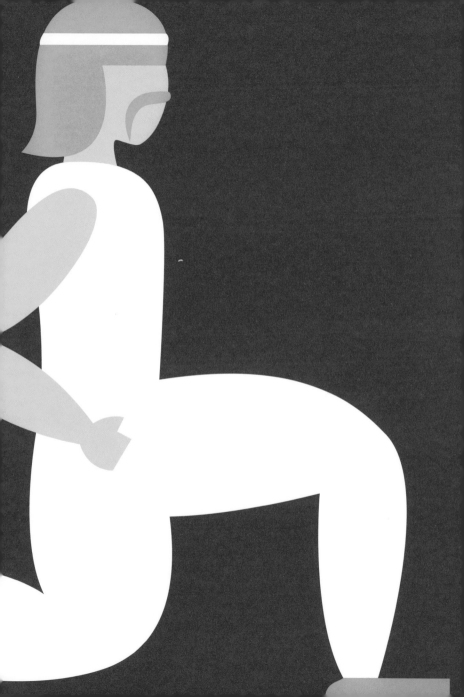

HELP IS
AT HAND

The aim of this book is to help you factor in some basic movements to stretch and strengthen your body during the course of your day. If you are office-based, there are numerous exercises that can be done at your desk, or even discreetly alongside it. If you have the opportunity or facilities, either in the office or at home, practise any of the floor-based exercises when you can. At the end of this section are suggestions on how to 'pick and choose' your own series of daily routines, in addition to any other regular exercise you may be taking, to keep you supple, strong and pain-free, whatever your age.

Remember, start gently and take it easy. This is not a competition – the only 'prize' is the improvement in your health. If in any doubt about your own capacity to do any of these exercises, please check with your doctor, physiotherapist or other health professional.

CONSTRUCTIVE REST POSITION

While many of these exercises can be done sitting or standing by your chair – and it's recommended that you stand and walk when you can – some exercises begin lying down in the 'constructive rest position'. For this position, lie flat on the floor, with your neck lengthened and chin gently tucked (with just enough space between your chin and chest for an imaginary orange), shoulders down and relaxed, arms loosely by your sides, knees bent (parallel and a hip's width apart) and your feet flat on the floor.

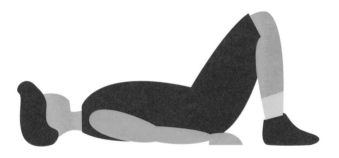

CORE MUSCLES

An important part of exercising is when we 'engage our core muscles' to strengthen and stabilise our bodies, protecting our backs and providing something of a power base for the whole body.

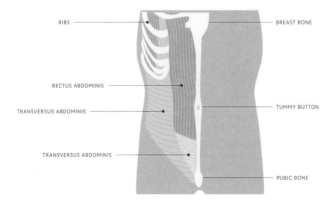

RIBS
BREAST BONE
RECTUS ABDOMINIS
TRANSVERSUS ABDOMINIS
TUMMY BUTTON
TRANSVERSUS ABDOMINIS
PUBIC BONE

Your core muscles consist of your *rectus abdominis* – the 'abs' that form your 'six pack' but also, importantly for stability, your *transverse abdominis* which wrap around the core of your body and lower down, just above the pubic bone. You can locate these muscles just above your pubic bone, and feel them working by doing a pelvic floor squeeze (page 81) while resting the tips of your fingers on the lower belly at the same time, and consciously tighten the muscles there. This is the area of muscular activity which is referred to as, 'engaging your core muscles', and means exactly that. If you activate your core muscles to 100 per cent and then release until 30 per cent *engagement*, that's the level of muscular activity you should experience when your core muscles are engaged.

Engaging your core muscles prior to a specific exercise means just that: engage those muscles so that they can support your back during the exercise. Keeping these muscles strong and engaged at 30 per cent all the time helps protects backs, supports your overall posture and keeps your tummy looking trim!

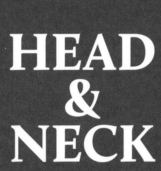

HEAD
&
NECK

The neck consists of seven bones, called the cervical vertebrae, on which the base of the skull sits. The neck is supported by a series of muscles attached to the base of the skull, one of which – the trapezius muscle – runs down over the shoulder (see diagram below); a large supportive ligament that is attached to the back of the skull and every cervical vertebrae; and the tendons, which connect the muscles to the bones.

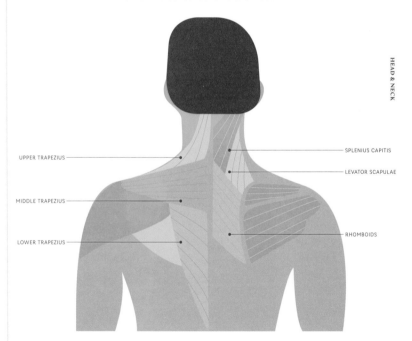

UPPER TRAPEZIUS

MIDDLE TRAPEZIUS

LOWER TRAPEZIUS

SPLENIUS CAPITIS

LEVATOR SCAPULAE

RHOMBOIDS

Long hours spent sitting at a computer, driving for long distances, bent over a smart phone, or slumped watching television, all take their toll on the neck. Why is this significant? Because the neck has to support the head, which is *heavy*. An adult's head weighs on average between 4.5–5 kg (10–12 lb). That's between three to four bags of flour – try holding those in your outstretched hand and see how long it is before your arm begins to ache! What's more, if your posture is poor and your head extends forward on your neck by just 15 degrees, the weight of your head increases to 12 kg (27 lb); by 30 degrees to 18 kg (40 lb); by 45 degrees to 22 kg (49 lb); and by 60 degrees to 27 kg (60 lb) of pressure on the neck. Unless we are vigilant, and check our posture, we tend to do this habitually as we look down to type, or hunch over our phones texting. This causes enormous strain on the muscles, tendons and ligaments in our necks, and also puts extra pressure on the vertebrae that these are trying to support.

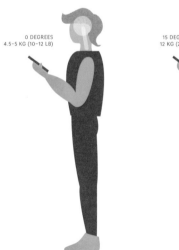

0 DEGREES
4.5–5 KG (10–12 LB)

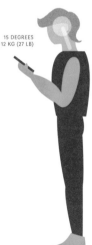

15 DEGREES
12 KG (27 LB)

The upshot of all this strain on the neck can be – unsurprisingly – chronic pain, not just in the neck but also in the shoulders and upper back, as they try to compensate for the extra weight. Persistent headaches, and even migraines, can be a direct consequence of the muscular strain that radiates from the base of the skull over the scalp to the forehead. It's that 'tense, nervous headache' beloved of pain-relief advertisers. If the muscles of your neck are strained and tense, this will affect the nerves of your head and cause the pain of a headache.

Gently exercising the neck not only relieves strain, tension and stiffness around the vertebral joints, it will also help to strengthen the muscles of the neck. Stronger neck muscles are more able to keep the head upright and supported in a good position; they are enabled to do the job they are meant to do in supporting the head, which relieves the pressure on the tendons and ligaments of the neck, reducing strain and the tired, achy pain that can arise.

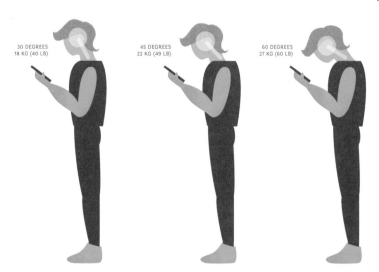

30 DEGREES
18 KG (40 LB)

45 DEGREES
22 KG (49 LB)

60 DEGREES
27 KG (60 LB)

Throughout this book, you may find references to 'keeping the neck long', particularly with regard to your overall posture or prior to doing an exercise. This refers to the position of your head and is the opposite of the 'poking chin posture', which is characteristic of working at a computer where the screen is set too high; or when you're trying to read the screen through the lower portion of varifocal glasses; or when your chair is too low. To lengthen the neck, you need to draw the chin in while lengthening the muscles in the back, finding its optimum, relaxed position.

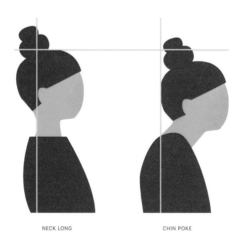

NECK LONG CHIN POKE

The
Exercises

Chin Tuck

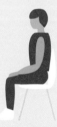

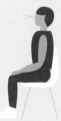

1 Sit upright in your chair, with your legs uncrossed, knees hip-width apart and feet flat on the floor.

2 Relax your shoulders and rest your hands in your lap.

3 Look ahead, with your chin tucked in, so that the back of your head is in line with your back (page 28).

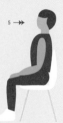

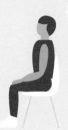

5x

4 Pull your chin in, keeping your gaze level, as if you were trying to press the back of your head against a wall.

5 Hold for a count of 5.

6 Relax.

7 Repeat 5 times.

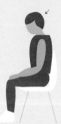

8 You can also extend this stretch by looking down, as if you were going to press your chin into your breastbone.

Forward Neck Flex

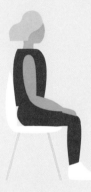

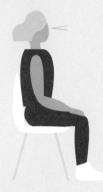

1 Sit upright in your chair, with your legs uncrossed, knees hip-width apart and feet flat on the floor.

2 Relax your shoulders and rest your hands in your lap.

3 Look ahead, with your chin tucked in, so that the back of your head is in line with your back.

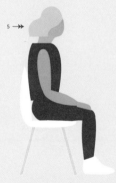

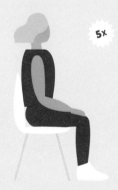

4 Keeping your shoulders down and relaxed and your head level, move your chin forwards.

5 Hold for a count of 5.

6 Relax.

7 Repeat 5 times.

Simple Neck Stretch

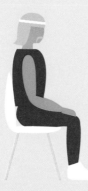

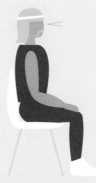

1 Sit upright in your chair, with your legs uncrossed, knees hip-width apart and feet flat on the floor.

2 Relax your shoulders and rest your hands in your lap.

3 Look ahead, with your chin tucked in, so that the back of your head is in line with your back.

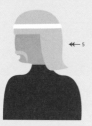

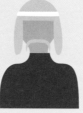

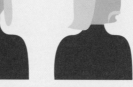

3x

4 Keeping your gaze level and your chest facing forward, turn your head to the right, until you feel the stretch in the opposite side of your neck. Don't over-extend or force your head round at this point – it's a gentle stretch. Remember, keep the shoulders relaxed.

5 Breathe gently as you hold the stretch, for a count of 5.

6 Return your head to the centre. Pause to check your posture. Repeat on the other side.

7 Repeat this sequence 3 times.

Extended Neck Stretch

This is an extension of the
Simple Neck Stretch (exercise 3, opposite).

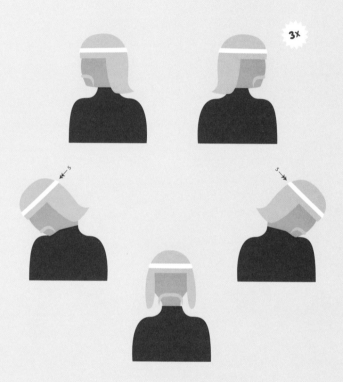

1 This time, when you have turned your head to the right, instead of holding the stretch in this position, look down to your right shoulder and hold for a count of 5.

2 Return your head to the centre position; repeat on the left side.

3 Repeat this sequence 3 times.

Lying
Neck Stretch

A variation of the Simple Neck Stretch (exercise 3, page 32) can be done lying on the floor. This ensures that your head is in a good position and is supported, while you allow the muscles, tendons and ligaments a gentle and passive stretch.

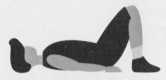

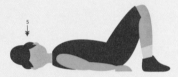

1 Lie on the floor in the Constructive Rest Position (page 22).

2 Using the weight of your head, allow it to roll first to the right and hold for a count of 5.

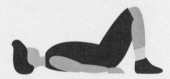

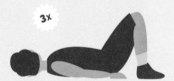

3x

3 Return your head to the centre; repeat on the other side.

4 Repeat this sequence 3 times.

5 Again, the Simple Neck Stretch can progress to the Extended Neck Stretch (exercise 4, page 33) while lying on the floor.

Gentle Neck Rotation

Having gently taken your neck through the preceding series of exercises, helping to wake and stretch the muscles, it's time to relax and loosen everything with a series of small, gentle neck rotations.

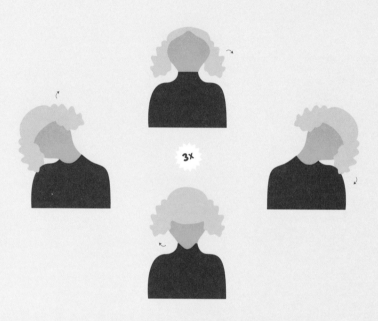

3x

1 Gently rotate your head by looking down, looking right, circling up and round to look left and then down again.

2 Rotate 3 times in one direction; repeat 3 times in the other direction.

3 Relax.

4 Use this gentle rotation regularly to ease your neck during any time spent stationary in front of a computer, laptop or television screen.

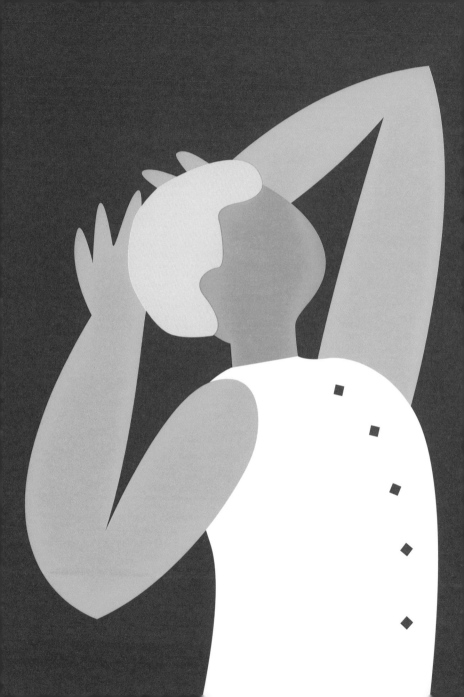

In addition to stretching the muscles, ligaments and tendons of the neck to ease tension and pain, strengthening the muscles will help support the head's weight and, in combination with good posture and regular gentle stretching, will help avoid the sort of strain that can lead to headaches and migraine. The simplest neck strengthening exercise uses just your own hands, to provide a bit of resistance against which to work (exercise 7, page 38).

Sitting
Resistance Exercise

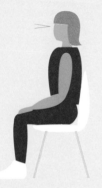
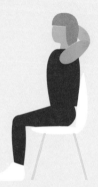

1 Sit upright in your chair, look straight ahead, knees hip-width apart and feet flat on the floor, core muscles engaged (page 23), shoulders relaxed and down.

2 Keeping your chin tucked and your neck long, place your hands on the back of your head with your fingers interlaced.

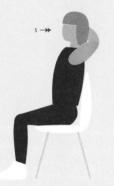
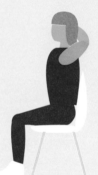

3 Gently push your head against your hands, holding firm while you do so, to feel the resistance and engagement in your neck muscles.

4 Hold for a count of 5; then relax.

5 Repeat, holding for a count of 10; then relax.

6 Repeat, holding for a count of 15; then relax.

7 Repeat the whole sequence.

Lying
Resistance Exercise

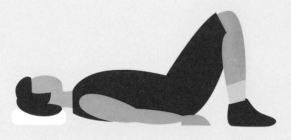

5,
10,
15
↓

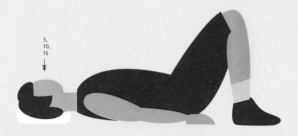

1 Instead of using your hands, you can do the same exercise lying in the Constructive Rest Position (page 22). Use a slim cushion or exercise mat to afford you some protection against a hard floor.

2 Repeat the whole sequence opposite, but gently push against the resistance of the floor, rather than your hands, to engage your neck muscles.

Lying
Neck Strengthening

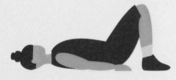

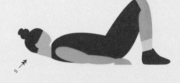

1 This is done lying on the floor in the Constructive Rest Position (page 22).

2 Without extending the chin, and keeping the neck long and shoulders relaxed and flat on the floor, raise your head from the floor just enough to feel the muscles of the neck engage.

3 Hold for a count of 5; then relax.

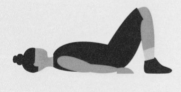

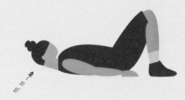

4 Repeat, holding for a count of 10; then relax.

5 Repeat, holding for a count of 15; then relax.

6 Repeat the whole sequence.

Lying Neck Strengthening, Prone

1 This time, lie on your tummy, with your arms bent in a diamond shape, so that your forehead is resting on the back of your hands.

2 Keeping the head in this position and with the neck long, gently raise your head a small distance above your hands. You should feel the muscles in your neck engage, rather than those in your shoulder.

3 Hold for a count of 5; then relax.

4 Repeat, holding for a count of 10; then relax.

5 Repeat, holding for a count of 15; then relax.

6 Repeat the whole sequence.

UPPER
BACK
&
SHOULDERS

Very often, it is on the shoulders that a lot of tension and stress will rest, even if the pain and discomfort is played out somewhere else in the body, perhaps in the arms or neck. Of course, all parts of the body are linked – some more closely than others. The shoulders and upper back link to the neck, the arms and the lower back, so keeping them strong will also support you elsewhere.

There are some very powerful, but often underused, muscles in the upper back, too, and these shouldn't be forgotten, especially when much of our sedentary work relies on them to support the arms and the neck. The trapezius muscle (page 25), for example, sits either side of the spine and runs from the middle of the back, over the shoulder and up into the neck. Tucked under the trapezius, attached to the shoulder blade, are the rhomboid muscles, which with a variety of other muscles all work towards supporting that heavy head (page 25). We make huge demands on them every day, and it's easy to see that if they are weak or stiff, they can't do the job for which they were designed and will let you know this through the discomfort and pain experienced. It really helps to pay attention to these powerful, under-appreciated muscles.

> All of the following exercises, apart from no. 5, 9 and 10, can be done either standing or sitting, but make sure that for each one your body is in good alignment: shoulders relaxed and down, neck long and chin tucked in, abdominal muscles engaged (page 23), and feet flat on the floor.

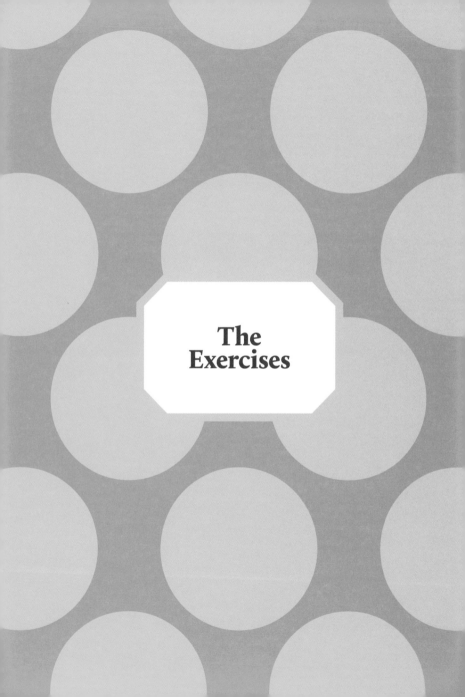

The
Exercises

Straight-Arm Shoulder Stretch

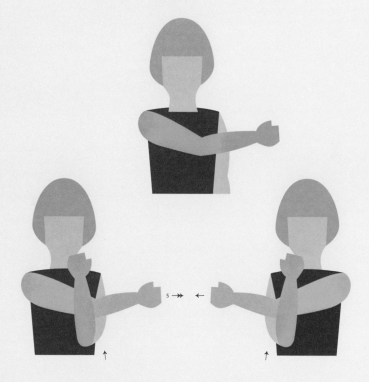

1 Working first with your left arm, reach forwards and across your body, with your arm at shoulder level.

2 Bend your right arm around the upper arm of your left, tucking your straight left arm into the crook of your right elbow.

3 Use the strength of your right arm to gently pull your left across your body. You should feel the stretch through your trapezius muscle, and also those around your shoulder blade.

4 Hold for a count of 5.

5 Release and repeat.

6 Alternate arms and repeat the sequence.

Bent-Arm Shoulder Stretch

This is similar to the Straight-Arm Stretch, (exercise 1, page 45)
but can be used as an alternative, with the previously straight arm,
bent at the elbow. This will increase the stretch through
the muscles of the rib cage a little more.

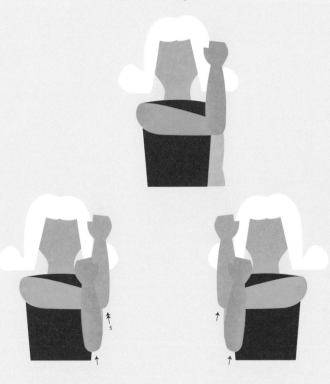

1 Hold for a count of 5.

2 Release and repeat.

3 Alternate arms and repeat the sequence.

Hugging Shoulder Stretch

Sometimes called the 'wrap-around stretch', this is effectively hugging yourself to create a stretch through the shoulder blades.

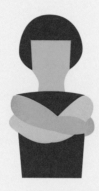
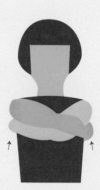

1 Once in this position, raise both elbows to shoulder height to gently increase the stretch.

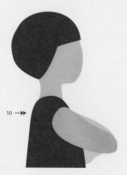
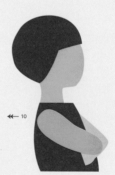

2 Now, gently move the shoulders forward in a hugging action and then back, to a count of 10.

3 Relax and repeat.

Cactus Position Shoulder Stretch

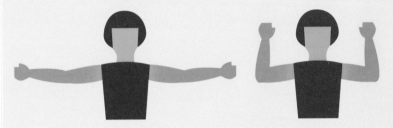

1 Raise both arms to the side at shoulder level.

2 Bend your arms upwards at the elbow, so your forearm is at right angles to your upper arm, palms facing forwards, as if you were a policeman halting traffic.

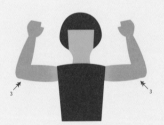

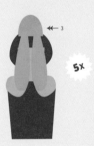

5x

3 In this 'cactus' position, gently push back, to activate the muscles between your shoulder blades and spine, and hold for a count of 3.

4 Now, round your shoulders, bring your arms to your front, and line your forearms up against each other – elbows, arms, wrists and palms touching – in a 'prayer' position.

5 Hold for a count of 3.

6 Repeat this sequence 5 times.

Reverse Shoulder Stretch

This is probably easier to do standing, rather than sitting.

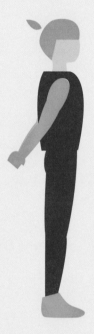
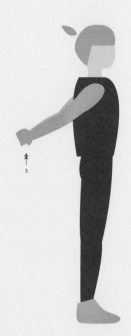

1. Clasp your hands behind your back.

2. Keeping your arms straight, slowly lift your clasped hands, so you feel the stretch at the front of your shoulders and through your biceps.

3. Hold for a count of 5.

4. Relax and repeat.

Shoulder Shrugging

This exercise targets and strengthens
your trapezius muscle.

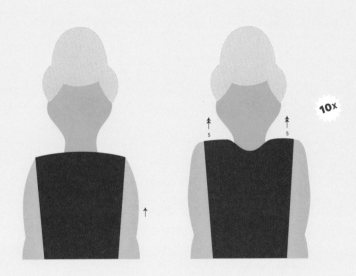

1 Leave your arms relaxed by your sides.

2 Raise your shoulders as high as you can,
as if you were trying to touch your ears.

3 Hold for a count of 5, then relax.

4 Repeat 10 times.

Shoulder Roll

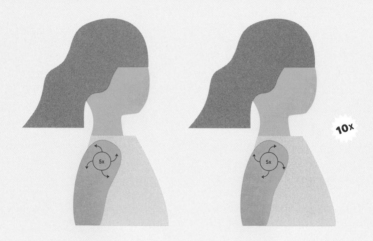

1 With your arms relaxed and by your sides, rotate your shoulders up towards the ears, forwards, down and back in circles.

2 Repeat 5 times in one direction, then rotate up, backwards, down and forwards in the other direction.

3 Repeat this sequence 10 times.

Shoulder Squeeze

This will also help strengthen your upper back.

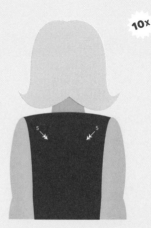

1 Leave your arms relaxed by your sides.

2 Squeeze your shoulder blades together as hard as you can without causing discomfort, but so you can feel the upper back muscles engage.

3 Hold for a count of 5, then relax.

4 Repeat the sequence 10 times.

Lying Body Stretch (1)

Probably not one for the office, but, whenever you can, a full body stretch not only feels good but helps body alignment, too.

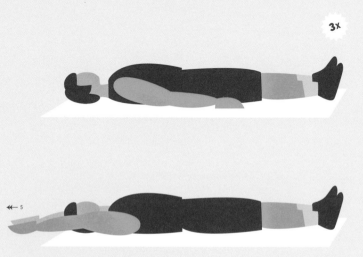

1. Lie on the floor, with an exercise mat or rug beneath you.

2. Your legs need to be straight out in front of you for this exercise, rather than in the Constructive Rest Position (page 22), but if this is uncomfortable for your lower back at first, keep the knees a little bent. Either way, you will need to engage your core abdominal muscles (page 23).

3. With your neck long and the back of your head on the floor, make sure that your shoulders are square to the floor, then gently lift your straight arms over your head to rest backwards on the floor behind you, palms facing up.

4. When you first do this, you may find that your shoulders are stiff and your arms don't want to lie flat. Be gentle with your shoulders, easing into position without forcing beyond what's comfortable.

5. Avoid reaching back and flaring your rib cage: the stretch should be felt through your upper back muscles not your stomach. Engaging your core muscles and pulling in with these should help, too.

6. Hold for a count of 5, then relax.

7. Repeat 3 times.

Lying
Body Stretch
(2)

As an alternative, and to ease through the shoulders, you
can gently scissor the arms (taking one back at a time then
alternating), keeping them straight, for a count of 20.

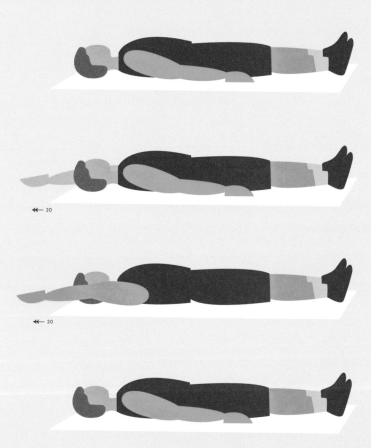

←← 20

←← 20

Kneeling Forward Stretch

Those familiar with yoga will recognise this as Child's Pose, but with the arms stretched out in front.

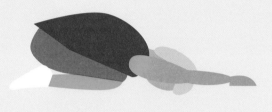

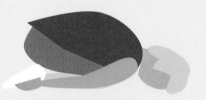

1 Kneel on the floor, with either your knees together or slightly apart, to ensure the bend can come from the hips and the stretch through the upper back.

2 Lean forward, with your arms stretched out in front.

3 If this is at all uncomfortable in your arms, keep them soft and the elbows slightly bent, ensuring that the stretch comes from the upper back, not the shoulders.

4 Hold the position for a count of 20, or however long you find comfortable.

5 It can also be nice to do this at the end of a series of exercises, drawing the arms in or to the sides, using Child's Pose as a rest position.

ARMS

When it comes to sitting and the damage it can do to our bodies, why should having strong arms be important? It's not just the sitting that's relevant here, but what we do when we're sitting for long hours; many of us are using a keyboard. Holding our arms in one position, making micro-movements with our hands, is stressful and tiring on the body and can give rise to Repetitive Strain Injury (RSI). If the muscles in our arms are strong, however, they do the work they were designed to do and this reduces the strain on the tendons and ligaments. Without strong muscles in the arms our body isn't fully supported; the shoulders tend to rotate and slump forwards, pulling on the upper back and causing problems there, too.

The great thing about your arms is that you can use their own weight to do quite simple exercises, which are very effective. Then, when you've become familiar with them and devised your own routine (page 109), you can take the exercises up a notch, by using either light, hand-held weights or even a can of beans from the kitchen cupboard. In some exercises, a resistance exercise band is used – this is easy to keep by your workstation, at home or in the office. The exercises outlined here are designed to strengthen the muscles in the arms and, in some cases, to provide a gentle stretch through the joints, because tight ligaments and tendons can also contribute to discomfort and pain.

It's worth becoming familiar with all these exercises, but you don't have to do them all, every time, or for the length of time or number of repetitions suggested. Always start gently and get a sense of what your body responds to and build on that, rather than force it too quickly. Mix and match these exercises, and combine with others (pages 108–121), and work with what you feel your body needs.

The
Exercises

Forward Raise

You can do this either sitting in your chair or standing. Opt for standing, if you can, because it's easier to focus on your core and posture, which adds benefit to the exercise. If you sit, make sure your feet are flat on the floor, knees square, tummy tucked in and your posture upright and strong.

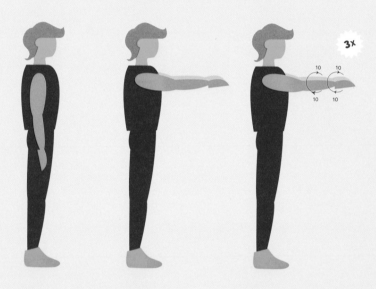

1 Make sure your shoulders are relaxed and down, engage your core muscles (page 23) and ensure your neck is long.

2 Keep your shoulders strong and square with your chest, then without reaching forwards and keeping both arms straight, raise your arms to shoulder height. Ensure you also keep the elbows and wrists soft.

3 Hold for a count of 10.

4 Holding this position, gently rotate the arms and hands from the shoulders, in small circles; repeat this 10 times alternating first clockwise then anticlockwise.

5 Relax the arms.

6 Repeat the sequence, always checking that your posture and the position of your shoulders is strong but relaxed before each repetition.

7 Start with a series of 3 repetitions, on which you can build.

Alternate Raise

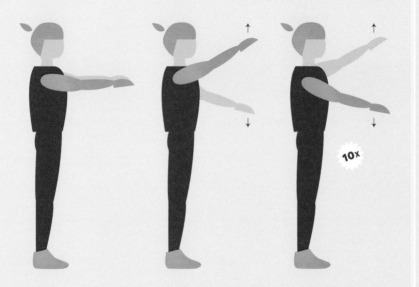

10x

1 As before, but this time, instead of rotating the arms, do a series of alternate straight arm raising and lowering, moving gently from the shoulder, keeping the raise no more than 30 cm (12 in) above and below the shoulder line.

2 Repeat 10 times.

3 Relax the arms.

Sideways Raise

This is probably easier to do standing. Make sure your feet are flat on the floor, legs hip-width apart, with a strong core and tummy muscles tucked in, neck long and shoulders relaxed.

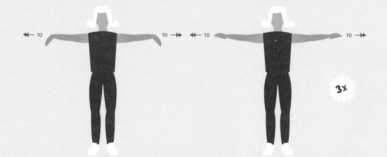

1 Raise your arms on either side to shoulder level, keeping palms face down and elbows and wrists soft.

2 Hold for a count of 10.

3 Next, consciously engaging your muscles, stretch through the arms, extending all the way through to the fingertips, keeping the shoulders firm.

4 Hold for a count of 10.

5 Repeat 3 times.

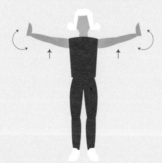

6 You can also extend the stretch further through the fingertips, if you like, by flexing the wrist and raising the hands up and down.

Arm Circle

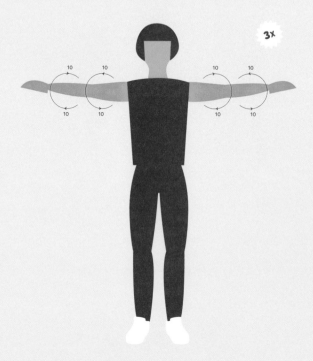

1 With your arms extended, either in front of you in a Forward Raise, or to the side in a Sideways Raise, smoothly rotate each arm, working from the shoulder, in small circles.

2 Rotate first one way for 10 circles, then in the other direction for a further 10 circles.

3 Repeat 3 times.

Small Weights (1)

You can use small, hand-held weights, cans of beans, small 500 ml (17 fl oz) bottles of water or a couple of hardback books of equal weight, one in each hand, depending on what you have available.

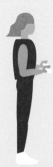

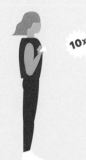

1 Stand or sit, with both feet firmly flat on the floor, in a good upright posture, with your core engaged (page 23) and the neck long. Your arms should be held at your sides from shoulder to elbow, and your forearms held in front at a right angle to your body, wrists rotated up, with a weight in each hand.

2 In this position, bring the weights up to your shoulders and down again, in a smooth movement; repeat 10 times.

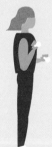

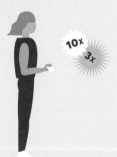

3 Then, alternate one arm bend with the other; repeat 10 times.

4 Repeat the sequence 3 times.

Small Weights (2)

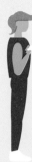
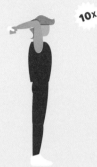

1 Position yourself as before, holding the weights in your hands.

2 This time, bend your elbows at right angles, so that your hands and weights are upright, wrists facing toward your body.

3 Next, lift both elbows up, as if you were going to pass the weights backwards over your shoulders.

4 Repeat this movement smoothly, pausing at the top of the lift for a beat or two; repeat 10 times.

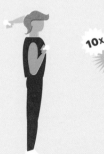

5 Next, alternate one arm with another; repeat 10 times.

6 Repeat the sequence 3 times.

Resistance Band Bicep Curl

For a similar effect to the exercises with small weights,
you can use a resistance band.

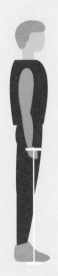

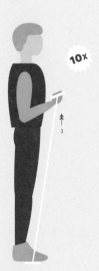

1 Stand upright, feet hip-width apart, and with your resistance band securely under one foot.

2 Grasp each end of the band, in each hand, at a length that provides you with some resistance: you can lengthen or shorten this in line with the amount of resistance you want.

3 Keeping your elbows at your sides, your shoulders relaxed and down, your posture strong and neck long, pull upwards from the elbows against the resistance of the band.

4 Hold for a count of 3, then release.

5 Repeat 10 times.

6 Remember, the movement, both as you pull against the resistance band and release, should be smooth and controlled.

Resistance Band Tricep Exercise

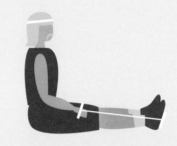

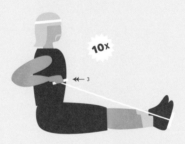

1 For this, you will need to sit on the floor in an upright position, shoulders square, core engaged (page 23), neck long, with sit bones firm to the ground and legs stretched out in front of you. Place the resistance band around your feet.

2 Pulling against the resistance, straighten your arms as you take them back behind, which activates the triceps.

3 Hold for a count of 3, then relax the arms.

4 Remember to keep the movements smooth and controlled.

5 Repeat 10 times.

Forearm stretch against wall

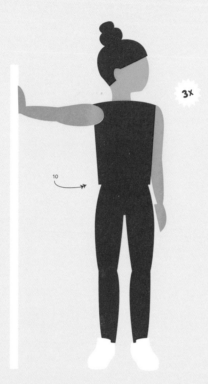

1 Stand with your arm at shoulder height, the palm of your hand against the wall.

2 Press lightly against the wall with your hand, then turn your body away from the wall, so that you can feel a gentle stretch through the chest, shoulder, upper arm and forearm.

3 Hold for a count of 10 then relax. repeat 3 times.

4 Repeat the sequence with the other arm.

Inner Forearm Stretch

This area of the arm can become quite foreshortened and weak. This stretch also provides a gentle, opposite stretch to the other arm exercises.

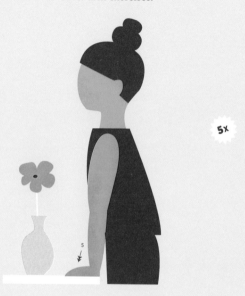

5x

1 Rest the heel of each hand on the edge of a desk or table and gently push down for a count of 5.

2 Release and repeat 5 times.

With any exercise sequence, check you aren't inadvertently holding your breath on exertion. Always ensure that you are mindful of your breathing, keeping it even during any exercise.

FINGERS,
HANDS
&
WRISTS

It would be a mistake, when exercising the arms, to leave out what's at the end of them, especially since there are many of us who spend long hours doing repetitive, manual work such as typing. You can use a hand-strengthening exercise ball, which is often used in treatment for RSI, tendonitis or carpel tunnel syndrome, to improve strength and dexterity, but here also are four quick exercises to add to your repertoire.

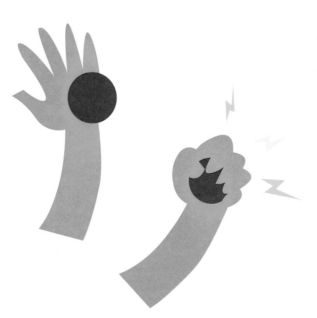

Prayer Stretch

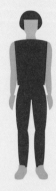

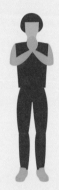

1 Keeping your shoulders square, relaxed and down, engage your core (page 23) without flaring your rib cage. Your body should be in good alignment, but relaxed, either sitting or standing, but with feet squarely on the floor.

2 Put your hands together, finger-to-finger, hands pointing upwards.

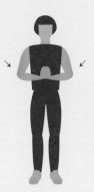

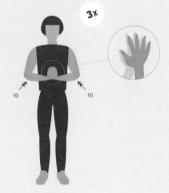

3x

10   10

3 Bend your elbows, so your hands are gently pushing against each other, with your wrists at right angles to your arms.

4 Splay your fingers, stretching them apart, while pressing together; your thumbs should just touch your breastbone.

5 Hold for a count of 10, then pause and relax.

6 Repeat 3 times.

Forearm & Wrist Stretch (I)

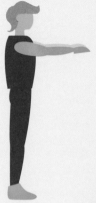

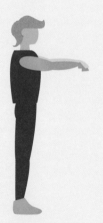

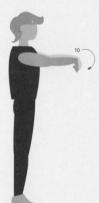

1 Standing or sitting, stretch your arms out in front of you.

2 With the palm of your right hand facing down, make a gentle fist and, curling your left hand around the fist, apply enough pressure with the left hand to help increase the stretch through the wrist and the top of the arm.

3 Hold for a count of 10.

4 Alternate arms and repeat on the other side.

Forearm &
Wrist Stretch
(2)

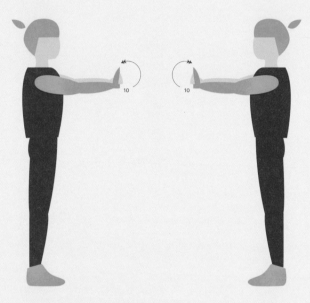

1 As in exercise 2, page 73, but this time keep the palm of the right hand turned upwards, use the fingers of your left hand to gently enhance the stretch the other way, for a count of 10.

2 Alternate hands and repeat on the other side.

Palms Out,
Forearm Stretch

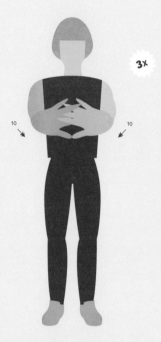

1 Keeping your shoulders square, relaxed and down, engage your core (page 23) without flaring your rib cage. Your body should be in good alignment, but relaxed, either sitting or standing, but with feet squarely on the floor.

2 Interlock your fingers together, then straighten your arms out in front of you, at shoulder height, turning the palms outwards.

3 Hold for a count of 10, then relax.

4 Repeat 3 times.

LOWER
BACK
&
BOTTOM

S itting for long periods slumped in a chair places particular strain on the lower vertebrae of the back, while those unused muscles in the abdomen and buttocks become weak and provide little support; all of which can create lower back pain, or aggravate chronic problems.

There is – believe it or not – even something called 'gluteal amnesia', a term coined by low back pain expert, Dr Stuart McGill, for the problems caused by weak buttock muscles. They're much more important than people realise – they provide the power to support the legs while walking, which supports the knee joints and helps to prevent that weakened, knock-kneed stance that causes problems in our walking gait. The buttock muscles, in conjunction with the abdominal muscles also support the lower back, keeping the pelvic girdle and hips in a good position.

Muscles of the buttocks

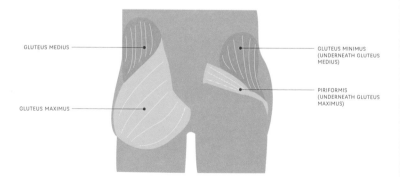

GLUTEUS MEDIUS

GLUTEUS MINIMUS
(UNDERNEATH GLUTEUS
MEDIUS)

PIRIFORMIS
(UNDERNEATH GLUTEUS
MAXIMUS)

GLUTEUS MAXIMUS

The following exercise sequences take you through a series of movements, designed to ease and strengthen your lower back. You can do as few or as many exercises as you wish, and alternate different options. Some exercises require more room or floor space, while others can be done either in your chair or alongside it. As you become familiar with these exercises, you can mix and match them as you like, but the key is to do whatever you choose *regularly*. Even 10 minutes of exercise, once a day, will make a difference, and on this you can build your own effective, daily routine (page 108). Never push yourself beyond what feels OK – done regularly, gentle stretching and strength building will be enough to ease most discomfort from extended hours spent sitting.

It is easier to sit upright if your posture is strong and this requires good abdominal muscles (page 23). Your posture will also be helped if your chair and desk are at the right height (page 15) – this will enable you to sit with your feet square and grounded on the floor. Avoid sitting with your legs crossed, too, as this will cause a twist through your body, which exacerbates muscular strain.

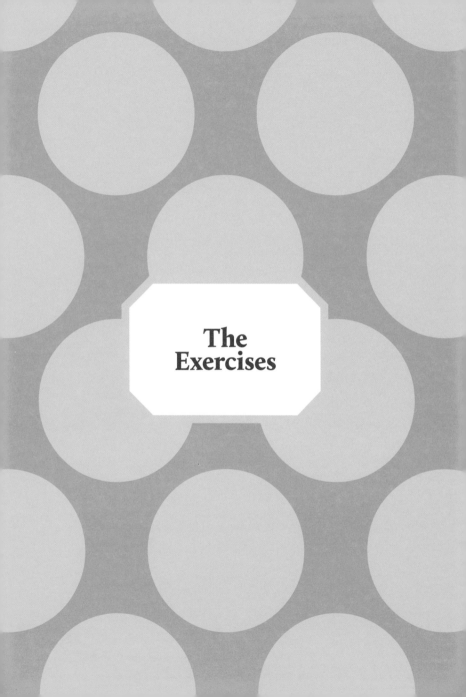

The Exercises

Buttock Clench

Even while sitting at your desk, buttock clenches are one of the easiest exercises you can do. They will not only strengthen the muscles of your bottom, to support your lower back, but will also improve circulation in this area.

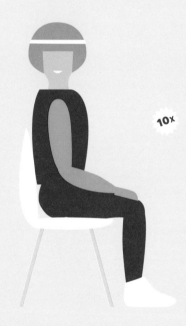

1 Sit square on your chair with your feet flat on the floor.

2 Deliberately tense and hold the muscles in your buttocks for a count of 10.

3 Release and repeat 10 times.

4 Aim to do this several times a day.

Pelvic Floor
Squeezes

Include pelvic floor squeezes along with your buttock clenches. These are important for both women and men, and can help guard against urinary incontinence in later life.

Locate your pelvic floor muscles in the way you would if you were trying to stop yourself peeing mid-stream.

Activate these internal muscles, 'pulling upwards', and hold to a count of 5, then release.

As you become more proficient, imagine your muscles as if they were an elevator travelling upwards, stopping at each of the floors on the way up. Pause briefly and hold at each 'floor'. Then 'descend' this muscular activity in the same way.

Exerting this sort of subtle control over these muscles will exercise and strengthen them more effectively.

Gentle Backward Stretch

Again, sitting in your chair, you can extend the buttock clench into a gentle backward stretch.

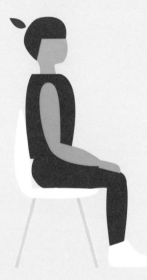
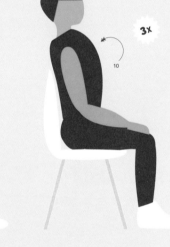

1 Sit square, with your feet flat on the floor.

2 Clench the buttocks and sit tall, with relaxed shoulders and hands gently resting on your lap.

3 Breathe in deeply and engage your core muscles, lift the chest up and lean back, stretching up and out from the waist. Keep the hips strong and grounded in your chair.

4 Hold for a count of 10 then relax: repeat 3 times.

Standing Backward Stretch

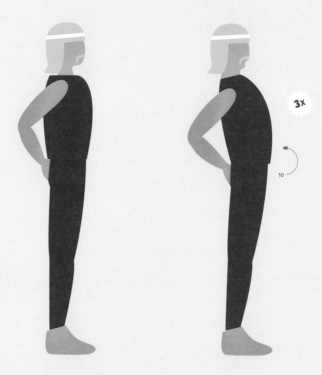

1 Alternatively, this gentle backward stretch can be done standing, with hands gently placed on your hips.

2 If you do this in the standing position, remember to tilt the pelvis a little up and in so that your abdominal muscles are engaged (page 23), for a more comprehensive stretch. Remember to *breathe* into the stretch.

3 Again, hold for a count of 10 then relax: repeat 3 times.

Lunge

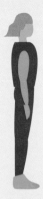 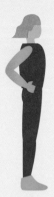

1 Stand with your feet well grounded, your tummy tucked in and shoulders relaxed.

2 Place your hands on your hips, keeping the hips square and facing forwards.

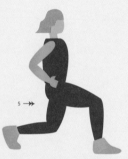

3 Breathe in and take a big step forward. Keep the knee of this leg at a right angle to your foot and in line with your big toe (this will protect your knees).

4 Keep your other leg extended in a line behind you, on the toes.

5 Dip the hips, to feel a gentle stretch through the muscles of the back of your waist at the top of your buttocks, and also the muscles of your thighs.

6 Hold for a count of 5. Then step the extended leg back.

7 Alternate right and left legs and build up to a sequence of 5 per side.

Piriformis
Stretch
(1)

The little piriformis muscle is buried deep in your buttock (see diagram on page 77) and can become very tight with prolonged sitting, which will, in turn, pull and create tension in other areas. This can lead to low back pain and even sciatica (when the pull on the sciatic nerve causes pain down the leg). The simplest way to ease this, and avoid problems, is with a series of stretches done lying flat on your back, on the floor.

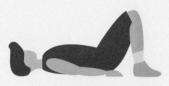

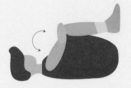

1 Start by lying comfortably on your back in the Constructive Rest Position (page 22).

2 Hug both knees to your chest and gently rock your hips from side to side. (This is also a good intermediate exercise, in between other floor-based exercises, to ease out the muscles of the back.)

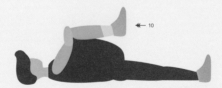

3 Stretch out one leg flat along the floor, while pulling the knee of the other leg in towards your chest, using both hands. Aim to feel a stretch through the buttock of the bent leg. Hold for a count of 10, then release and alternate sides.

4 Repeat on the other side.

Piriformis Stretch (2)

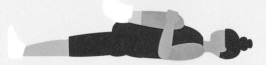

1 As in exercise 5, page 85, but this time, instead of pulling the knee in towards the chest, don't bend it so far but use the opposite arm and hand to draw that leg from the hip across the body. Aim to keep the other arm relaxed and resting on the floor, providing a little counter-balance, so that the stretch is felt in the buttock.

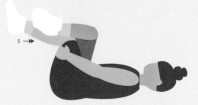

2 Now cross your legs and bend your knees in this cross-legged position. Loop your hands around the inner knee of the bottom leg and gently increase the pull of both legs towards your chest. Again, you should feel a strong stretch through the top of the buttock muscles.

3 Hold for a count of 5.

4 Repeat with the other leg.

Piriformis Stretch (3)

Do this stretch sitting in your chair.

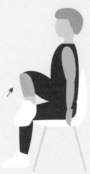

1 Keeping one foot flat and grounded on the floor, bend the other knee and place your ankle across the thigh of the opposite leg. The higher up your thigh, the greater the stretch, but start with what feels most comfortable, especially in the knee of the bent leg.

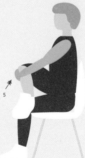

2 Holding the bent knee with both hands, and keeping your shoulders relaxed and back straight, gently pull up from the hips to increase the stretch from your buttock through the thigh of the bent leg.

3 Hold for a count of 5.

4 Repeat with the other leg.

Two-Knee Twist

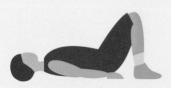

1 Lying on your back on the floor, start from the Constructive Rest Position (page 22).

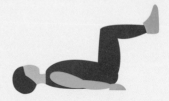

2 This time, bring your feet and knees together, and lift your knees towards your chest, 90° to your hips.

5x

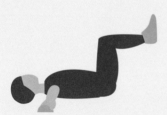

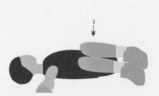

3 Keeping your shoulders in good contact with the floor, spread your arms wide in a 'T' shape.

4 Now, engage your stomach muscles (page 23) to protect your back and gently lower your knees to one side, keeping your shoulders on the floor.

5 When you first do this, you may not be able to lower your knees very far before your shoulders start to lift, so do not force your knees beyond this point, otherwise you will lose the stretch through the buttocks. It's better to lower only to the point where your alternate shoulder starts to lift.

6 Hold for a count of 3, then return your knees to the centre.

7 Alternate sides, completing a couple of repetitions if you can, and building up over time to 5 repetitions.

Cobra Stretch

This is a yoga exercise, designed to stretch and strengthen through the back of your waist and lower back.

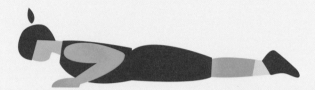

1 Lie flat on your stomach, elbows bent and hands flat on the floor at the shoulders, so you can raise your chest and rest on your forearms. Keep the elbows tucked towards the body and your upper arms in a straight line from your shoulders.

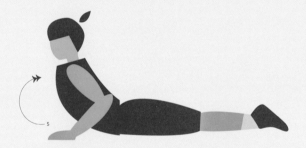

2 Although the lift is in the chest, consciously stretch up through the back of the waist into the front of the chest, easing the lower back. Press down gently into the thighs and top of the feet.

3 Hold for a count of 5; remember to breathe evenly and deeply through the stretch.

4 Relax the posture, pause and repeat.

Bridge

This is one of those exercises that is immediately effective and, even if tricky at first, easy to build on. It activates and strengthens your core muscles, buttock muscles and thigh muscles, all of which help support your posture.

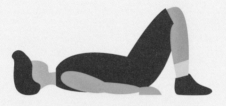

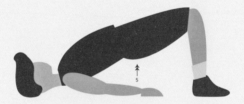

1 Lie on your back, with your knees bent and feet flat on the floor. You can do this exercise either with your knees together or a couple of inches apart.

2 Relax your neck by tucking your chin in a little, keep your shoulders square to the floor and your arms loosely by your sides with palms down.

3 Engage your abdominal core muscles (page 23) so that your pelvis curls up a little. Engage your buttock muscles and gently lift your hips up so that your body runs in a straight line from your shoulders to your knees.

4 Try to keep this movement as one, smooth curling up of the spine, almost as if you were lifting up one vertebra at a time.

5 Hold for a count of 5.

6 Gently release down – again, vertebra by vertebra. This rolling movement helps ease out the spine as you exercise.

7 Repeat.

With any floor-based exercise, take your time to return to a standing position, particularly if you have low-blood pressure and tend to feel dizzy. Make sure that you keep well hydrated too, drinking plenty of water after you've exercised.

LEGS

You may wonder what your legs might have to do with sitting strong, but they are as important as the rest of your body – and can get a bit neglected as a result of a sedentary lifestyle. If the muscles in your legs become weak from lack of use they can't do the job for which they were designed, keeping you upright and walking steady.

Quadricep and Hamstring Muscles

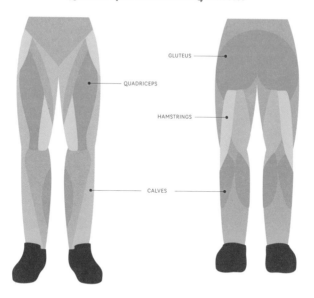

GLUTEUS

QUADRICEPS

HAMSTRINGS

CALVES

Front

Back

Your quads are the very strong muscles at the front of your thighs, and these are the ones that can really foreshorten from sitting. At the back of your thighs are the hamstrings. These muscles don't just enable walking, they also protect important joints, such as the knees. The knees take a lot of strain, and are consequently the most vulnerable of all the joints in the body. They need to be supported by the thigh muscles (the quadriceps at the front and the hamstrings at the back). If these muscles become weak from lack of use, the knee joints become more prone to injury.

If these muscles become foreshortened from sitting this, in turn, can cause problems by pulling on, and tilting, your pelvis out of alignment, which then affects the lumbar vertebrae of the spine. The result? As a consequence of sitting all the time, those strong, stabilising gluteus muscles at the top of your thighs become weak through 'gluteal amnesia' (page 77), which also makes you more prone to poor posture and backache.

Finally, remember that tricky little piriformis muscle (page 77)? The one that can cause so much pain and discomfort when it gets into trouble, by pulling on the sacroiliac joints of the back, tweaking that sciatic nerve and radiating pain down your leg? Stretching and strengthening your legs will help ease problems here as well, because all too often, back pain is linked to a weakness in the muscles of the legs.

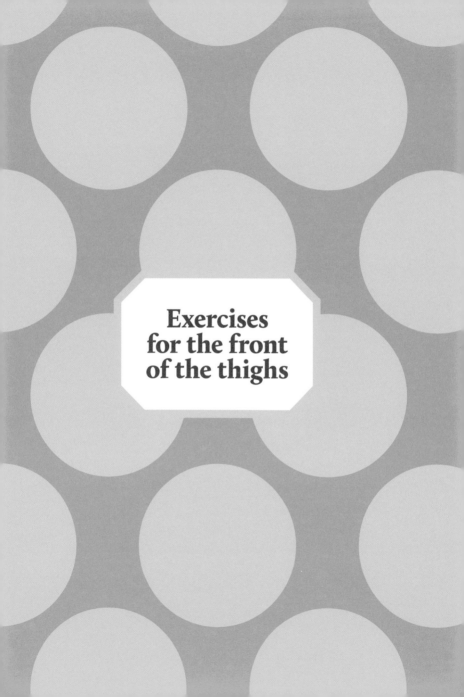

Exercises
for the front
of the thighs

Standing Quad Stretch

If you have problems with your knees,
you should undertake this exercise with care.

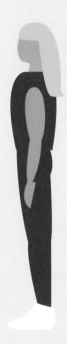
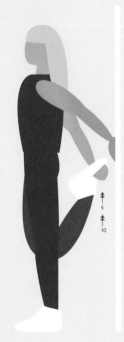

1 Stand with your feet pointing forward, hip-width apart, and with your hips, knees and ankles in alignment.

2 Engaging your core muscles (page 23), keeping your pelvis level, bend your right knee and lift your foot behind you, balancing on your left leg.

3 Reaching behind with your right hand, grasp your ankle.

4 If you need help to balance, align yourself against a wall to steady yourself with your left hand.

5 Hold the position for a count of 5, increasing to a count of 10 as you feel more confident.

6 Repeat on the other side.

Kneeling Quad Stretch

This is an alternative to the Standing Quad Stretch (exercise 1, opposite). If the floor is hard on the kneeling knee, place a folded rug underneath.

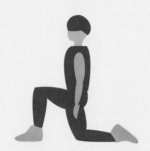

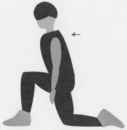

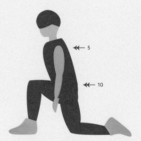

1 Kneel with one knee on the floor, and with the other leg bent at a right angle to your body. Ensure that your upper posture is aligned, your shoulders relaxed, and your core is engaged (page 23).

2 Leaning forwards a little into the bent leg, feel the stretch through the quad of the kneeling leg.

3 You can extend the stretch a little by pushing the hips forwards, but don't over-extend.

4 Hold for a count of 5, increasing to 10 as it feels beneficial.

5 Repeat on the other side.

Lying Quad Stretch

If you are comfortable lying on your stomach, you can try this.
It is the lying-down equivalent of the Standing Quad Stretch
(exercise 1, page 96). If you have problems with your knees,
you should undertake this exercise with care.

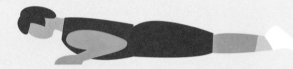

1 Lie on your stomach, with your upper body gently
raised on one forearm, and with both legs stretched
out behind you.

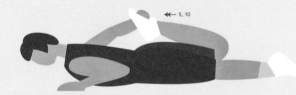

2 Bend your right leg up and, reaching round with
your right hand, grasp your ankle to extend the
stretch through the front of your thigh.

3 Hold the position for a count of 5, increasing to
a count of 10 as you feel more confident.

4 Repeat on the other side.

If you have problems with your knees, undertake
these exercises with care.

Exercises
for the back
of the thighs

Standing Hamstring Stretch – Toes Flat/Toes Raised

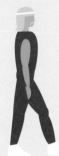

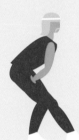

1 Stand with your feet pointing forwards, hip-width apart, and with your hips, knees and ankles in alignment, then step forwards with your right leg.

2 Bending your left knee, sink down, with a straight back, leaning into your right leg, resting both hands on the right thigh to steady yourself.

3 You should feel the stretch in the hamstrings of the right leg.

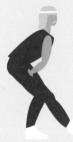

4 This exercise can be done first with the right foot flat, and then with the toes raised, on the heel.

5 You may find, at first, that your balance is a little unsteady until you are used to the exercise, so take it easy!

6 Once in position, hold for a count of 5, increasing to a count of 10 as you feel more confident.

7 Repeat on the other leg.

Lying Straight-
Leg Hamstring Stretch

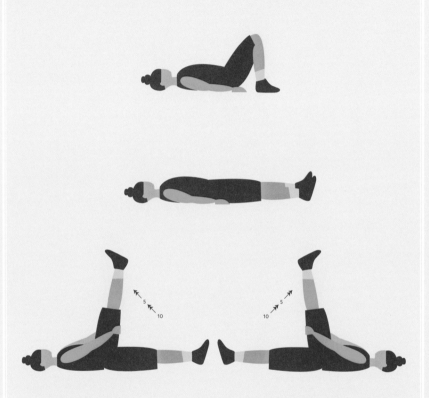

1 Lie on the floor, initially in the Constructive Rest Position (page 22), then straighten both legs, making sure your back is well supported by your core muscles.

2 Engage your core (page 23), and raise your right leg from the hip, keeping the knee straight but relaxed and your foot flat not pointed.

3 To increase and hold the stretch more comfortably, you can grasp your thigh with both hands and pull gently towards you.

4 Hold for a count of 5, increasing to a count of 10 as you feel more confident.

5 Repeat with the other leg.

Lying Bent-Leg Hamstring Stretch

This is the same exercise as before, but this time bend the knee of the raised leg, holding it with both hands. This will increase the stretch through the hamstring and the buttock muscle, and can be useful in releasing lower-back muscle stiffness.

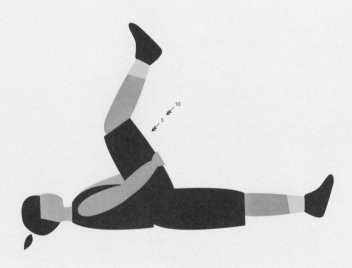

1 Hold for a count of 5, increasing to a count of 10 as you feel more confident.

2 Repeat with the other leg.

Standing Heel Calf Stretch

Perpetually wearing high heels will shorten the muscles in the calves, making them stiff and liable to ache. The Achilles tendon, which secures your calf muscle to your heel bone, can also become foreshortened and liable to injury. Regularly alternating the heel height of your shoes can help, as can the following exercises.

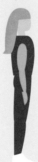

1 Stand with your feet pointing forwards, hip-width apart, and with your hips, knees and ankles in alignment.

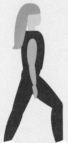

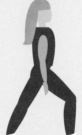

2 Engaging your core (page 23) and keeping your pelvis level, step forward with your right leg, bending into that knee. Keep your right knee aligned over the big toe on your right foot, and your left leg straight.

3 Push the heel of the left leg firmly into the ground as you lean forwards into the right leg, to feel the stretch in your calf.

4 Hold for a count of 5, increasing to a count of 10 as you feel more confident.

5 Repeat with the other leg.

Step
Calf Stretch

This is a very simple stretch,
but needs a step to work against.

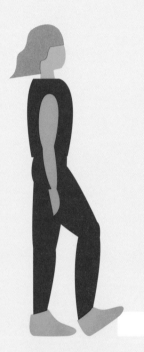
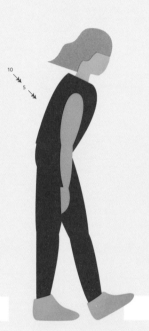

1 Standing a short stride away from the step, position your right foot with its heel at the base of the step, pressing your toes against it.

2 Keep your left leg straight and then lean into your right leg and foot, so you can feel a gentle stretch into your calf.

3 You can increase the stretch by leaning forward a little more, but take it easy at first.

4 Hold for a count of 5, increasing to a count of 10 as you feel more confident.

5 Repeat with the other leg.

Heel-Drop Stretches

Again, you need a step for this. You may need also to place your hand on a wall or stair rail for balance.

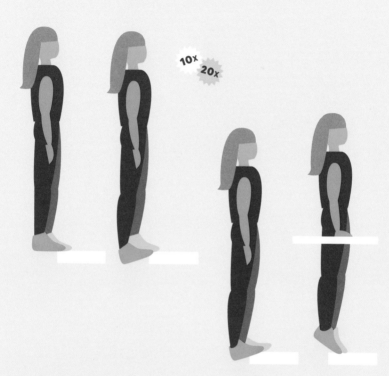

10x 20x

1 Stand with the balls and toes of both feet on the edge of the step, so that your heels are hanging over the edge.

2 Using your toes, and shifting your weight from one foot to the other, alternate lifting one heel up, while letting the other heel drop back down over the edge of the step.

3 Alternate 10 times, increasing to 20 as you gain strength and confidence.

4 You can also do this exercise without alternating, but by dropping both heels down, and then lifting up, together.

5 If you feel unsteady rest your hand on the wall or banister.

Straight-Leg, Roll-Down Stretch

This is a full body stretch, and one in which you can relax.
It stretches the hamstrings and the muscles through the back.
Throughout the stretch, keep your legs straight, your knees soft,
and arms relaxed, and use your body as a counter-weight to ease
your body forwards into the stretch.

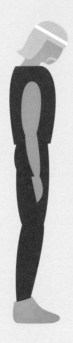
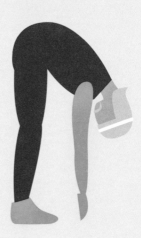
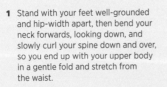

1 Stand with your feet well-grounded and hip-width apart, then bend your neck forwards, looking down, and slowly curl your spine down and over, so you end up with your upper body in a gentle fold and stretch from the waist.

2 Keeping the knees soft helps to extend the curve of the stretch through your back and into the muscles at the back of your legs.

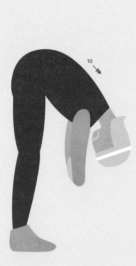

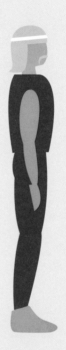

3 You can also fold your arms, grasping your elbows, to encourage your upper body to relax.

4 Hold for a count of 10, then slowly begin to uncurl until you are standing upright again.

PUTTING
IT
ALL
TOGETHER

Once you've worked your way through the suggested exercises and become familiar with them, and how they work from top to toe, you can work out your own personal routines. You can either devise a routine that focuses on one area, or move between them for a full body sequence, mixing and matching as your body needs.

Here are suggestions for some regular sequences that can be utilised as and when necessary – but regularly! – throughout the day. It's much better to do 10 minutes, even once or twice a day, than 40 minutes just once a week. Getting into the habit of doing them is key. And, remember, these are just suggestions – finding out what works best for you that means you are more likely to commit and do what you need to keep strong. Even if you do have to spend long hours sitting, you can counteract this through exercise.

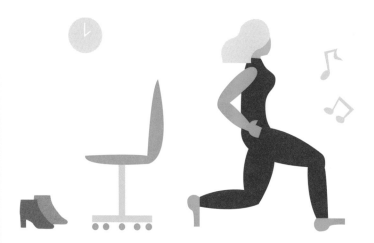

Head & Neck

This sequence can be done simply and regularly at any time and will remind you also to keep your sitting posture strong.

Simple Neck Stretch (page 32)

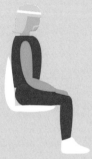 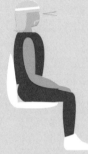 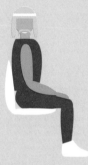

1 Sit upright in your chair, with your legs uncrossed, knees hip-width apart, and your feet flat on the floor.

2 Relax your shoulders and rest your hands in your lap.

3 Look ahead, with your chin tucked in, so that the back of your head is in line with your back.

4 Keeping your gaze level and your chest facing forwards, turn your head to the right, until you feel the stretch in the opposite side of your neck. Don't over-extend or force your head round at this point – it's a gentle stretch. Remember, keep the shoulders relaxed.

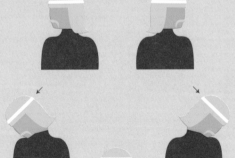

Extended Neck Stretch
(page 33)

7 Repeat the Simple Neck Stretch sequence, but instead of returning to the centre, continue the stretch through a gentle rolling movement, a couple of times.

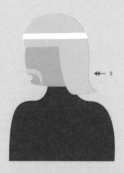

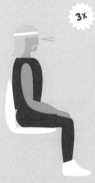

5 Breathe gently as you hold the stretch, for a count of 5.

6 Return your head to the centre. Pause to check your posture. Repeat on the other side. Repeat this sequence 3 times.

Chin Tuck (page 30)

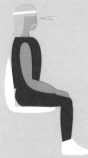

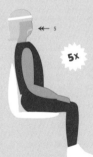

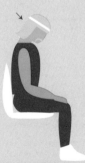

8 Look ahead, with your chin tucked in, so that the back of your head is in line with your back (page 28).

9 Pull your chin in, keeping your gaze level, as if you were trying to press the back of your head against a wall.

10 Hold for a count of 5.

11 Relax, and repeat 5 times.

12 You can also extend this stretch by looking down, as if you were going to press your chin into your breastbone.

Upper Body Sequence

Here's a sequence designed to activate your upper body.
You can do this sitting in a chair or standing, as you prefer.

Shoulder Roll (page 51) ### Simple Neck Stretch (page 32)

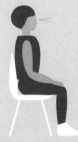 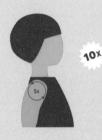 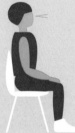

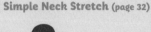

1 Sit upright in your chair, with your legs uncrossed, knees hip-width apart, and your feet flat on the floor.

2 Relax your shoulders and rest your hands in your lap.

3 With your arms relaxed, rotate your shoulders up, forwards, down and back in circles.

4 Repeat 5 times in one direction, then rotate up, backwards, down and forwards in the other direction.

5 Repeat this sequence 10 times.

6 Look ahead, with your chin tucked in, so that the back of your head is in line with your back.

Hugging Shoulder Stretch (page 47)

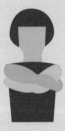 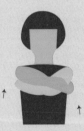

11 Sometimes called the 'wrap-around stretch', this is effectively hugging yourself to create a stretch through the shoulder blades.

12 Once in this position, raise both elbows to gently increase the stretch.

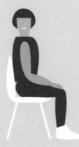

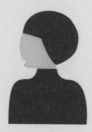

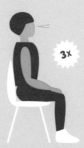

7 Keeping your gaze level and your chest facing forward, turn your head to the right, until you feel the stretch in the opposite side of your neck. Don't over-extend or force your head round at this point – it's a gentle stretch. Remember, keep the shoulders relaxed.

8 Breathe gently as you hold the stretch, for a count of 5.

9 Return your head to the centre. Pause to check your posture. Repeat on the other side.

10 Repeat this sequence 3 times.

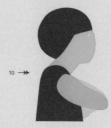

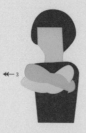

13 Now, gently move the shoulders forwards and then back, to a count of 10.

14 Relax and repeat.

15 Keeping the same position, gently rotate your upper body to the right and hold for a count of 3. Return to the centre, then repeat on the other side.

Sideways Raise (page 62)

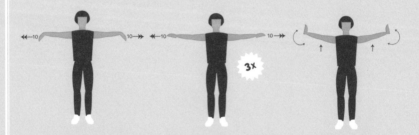

16 Raise your arms on either side to shoulder level, keeping the palms facing down and the elbows and wrists soft.

17 Hold for a count of 10.

18 Next, consciously engage your muscles and stretch through the arms, extending all the way through to the fingertips, keeping the shoulders firm.

19 Hold for a count of 10.

20 Repeat 3 times.

21 You can also extend the stretch further through the fingertips, if you like, by flexing the wrist and raising the hand at right angles to the arm.

Prayer Stretch (page 72)

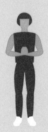
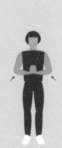
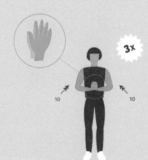

22 Put your hands together, finger-to-finger, hands pointing upwards.

23 Bend your elbows, so your hands are gently pushing against each other, with your wrists at right angles to your arms.

24 Splay your fingers, stretching them apart, while pressing together; your thumbs should just touch your breastbone.

25 Hold for a count of 10, then pause and relax.

26 Repeat 3 times.

Lower Body Sequence

Stand or sit with your body in good alignment, shoulders relaxed and down, neck long and chin tucked in, abdominal muscles engaged, legs hip-width apart, knees soft and feet grounded on the floor.

Buttock Clench
(page 80)

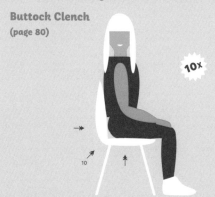

1 Deliberately tense and hold the muscles in your buttocks for a count of 10.

2 Relax and repeat 10 times.

Standing Backward Stretch (page 83)

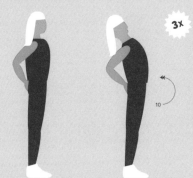

3 With hands resting on your hips, breathe in to your abdomen. Lifting the chest up, gently lean back, stretching up and out from the waist.

4 Hold for a count of 10.

5 Remember to *breathe* through the stretch. Repeat 3 times.

CONTINUE OVERLEAF >>

Lunge
(page 84)

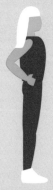

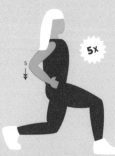

6 With your hands still on your hips, keeping the hips square and facing forwards, breathe in and take a big step forward. Keep the knee of this leg at a right angle to your foot and in line with your big toe (this will protect your knees).

7 Keep your other leg extended in a line behind you, on the toes. Dip the hips to feel a gentle stretch through the muscles of the legs and lower waist.

8 Hold for a count of 5.

9 Alternate right and left legs and repeat 5 times.

Straight-Leg, Roll-Down Stretch (page 106)

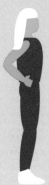

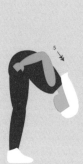

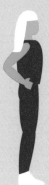

10 Standing as before, drop your chin, looking down, and curl your spine down and over, so you end up with your upper body in a gentle fold and stretch from the waist.

11 Keeping the knees soft helps to extend the curve of the stretch through your back and into the muscles at the back of your legs.

12 Hold for a count of 5, then slowly begin to uncurl, until you are standing upright again.

Full Body Sequence

If you put the first three sequences together, you will have a slightly longer – but comprehensive – sequence that takes you effectively through the whole body.

Relaxation Body Sequence

We all lead such busy lives that taking time to relax can easily be forgotten. Relaxing the body, through exercise, is also a way to relax the mind. By focusing on doing something physical, it can take you mind away from all those thoughts scurrying through your brain, jostling for attention. If you factor in your breathing, using that too to help you focus and relax, then you are maximising the potential for any series of stretching and strengthening exercises. This sequence takes this all into account and is designed to ease and relax your body. It is a useful sequence to do at the end of the day.

Start by lying comfortably on your back in the Constructive Rest Position (page 22). Take a moment to 'check in' with your body and adjust your breathing, as you relax.

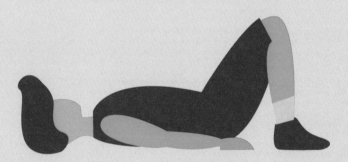

Lying Neck Stretch (page 34)

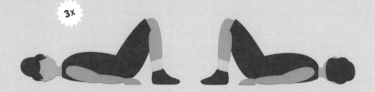

1 Using the weight of your head, allow it to roll to the right and hold for a count of 5, then return to the centre and do the same on the other side.

2 Repeat this sequence 3 times.

Two-Knee Twist (page 88)

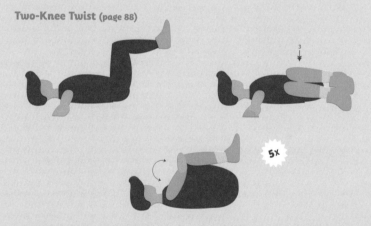

3 Bring your feet and knees together, and lift your knees towards your chest.

4 Keeping your shoulders in good contact with the floor, spread your arms wide in a 'T' shape. Engage your stomach muscles (page 23) and gently lower your knees towards one side, keeping your shoulders on the floor.

5 Only go as far as is comfortable and ensure your shoulders are still in good contact with the floor.

6 Hold for a count of 3, then return your knees to the centre.

7 Repeat on the other side. Alternate sides, completing a couple of repetitions if you can, and building up over time to 5 repetitions.

8 Follow this by hugging your knees in to your chest and rocking a little from side to side.

CONTINUE OVERLEAF >>

Lying Cactus Position Stretch (page 48)

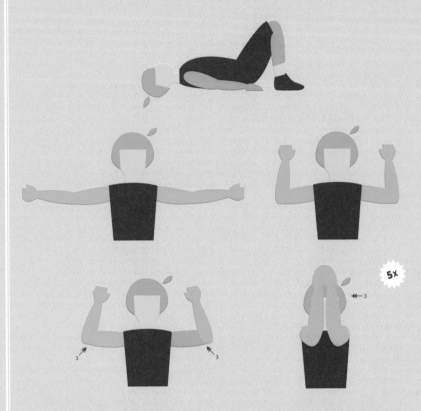

5x

9 Lie in the Constructive Rest Position (page 22). Spread your arms wide in a 'T' shape, keeping your shoulders relaxed and in good contact with the floor.

10 Bend your arms at the elbow, so your forearm is at right angles to your upper arm, palms facing forwards, with the back of your hand on the floor.

11 Holding this 'cactus' position, gently push back, to activate the muscles between your shoulder blades and spine, and hold for a count of 3.

12 Now, round your shoulders, bring your arms to your front, and line your forearms up against each other – elbows, arms, wrists and palms touching – in a 'prayer' position in front of your face.

13 Hold for a count of 3.

14 Repeat this sequence 5 times.

Lying Body Stretch (I) (page 53)

3×

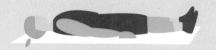

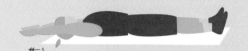

←— 5

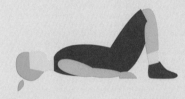

Kneeling Forward Stretch (page 55)

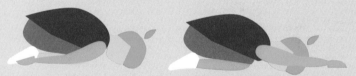

15 Stretch one leg out straight, then the other. Keep your stomach muscles engaged, so that there is good contact between the lower back and the floor.

16 Stretch one arm, and then the other, over your head, so you are reaching behind you.

17 Take a breath in and, as you breathe out, stretch through your whole body from your toes to your fingertips.

18 Hold for a count of 5, then relax.

19 Repeat 3 times.

20 Relax back in the Constructive Rest Position (page 22).

21 Alternatively, if you are comfortable on your knees, roll over to your front, kneel back on your heels and lean forward into Child's Pose (page 55), resting your forehead on the floor. Either stretch your arms out in front of you, or rest them alongside your thighs. You can have your knees splayed, if it's more comfortable. If your knees don't like it, take the pressure off by leaning over a large cushion, bolster or rolled-up rug.

Three.

WHAT
ELSE
HELPS
?

It's not just these strengthening and stretching exercises that will help you sit strong, you can also support this in a number of other ways, through other forms of specific exercise.

YOGA

Don't be put-off by the idea that you have to be very bendy and fit to do yoga – it's actually a form of exercise suitable for everyone. You can choose between a gentle and meditative Yin practice; a traditional Hatha form, with its focus on breathing work; or a more energetic Vinyasa style; but all yoga is based on strength-building and stretching postures that work with the breath. It may take a bit of research and a few trial classes to find what works best for you.

Yoga is something you can enjoy as a group activity, but you can also create a daily 10-minute practice for yourself, to do in your own home. It's a form of exercise that aims to restore a connection between the mind and body, so it has the added benefit of being calmly therapeutic, helping to turn down the stress thermostat, as well as building strength and flexibility. Check the training of any teacher offering classes and talk with them about what would be most appropriate for you.

PILATES

Pilates – named after Joseph Pilates, a physical trainer who originally worked with ballet dancers – is a particularly good way to improve your core stability and postural alignment. It works to improve muscle tone, whole body strength and stamina, through a series of exercises that work to balance both sides of the body. There's a lot of floor work and the use of exercise balls, instability 'wobble' boards, resistance bands and blocks, to help position the body during some of the exercises. Generally, attending a class, with an experienced and fully trained teacher is the best way to benefit, but many exercises can be integrated into your own practice.

There are various schools of training for Pilates teachers, including Body Control Pilates, so check your teacher is fully accredited and capable. Many Pilates teachers are also fully trained physiotherapists, which makes for a particularly good combination, as they really are body experts.

ALEXANDER TECHNIQUE

Devised by the actor Frederick Matthias Alexander in 1896, his original aim was to unlearn those poor postural habits that impeded his voice. The technique is a way to identify and prevent the harmful postural habits that aggravate, or may even be the cause of, stress, pain and under-performance. With the help of a teacher, practitioners of the technique learn how to release muscular tension, realign the body and help restore physical balance.

The idea is that, through increased bodily awareness, you can be poised without stiffness, move gracefully and powerfully with less effort, breathe more easily and generally calm your body and, through that, your mind. Improving patterns of posture and movement reduces the strain on the body, can alleviate pain and restore health.

T'AI CHI

T'ai chi originated as a Chinese martial art, but in the true tradition of its philosophy it trains the mind as well as the body. Its three key principles focus on physical health, through the relief of muscular tension and stress; meditation through the calmness of the physical movements; and self-defence, through yielding and responding rather than meeting it with an opposing force.

The sequence of movements and poses of t'ai chi is designed to balance internal energy but its slow-impact movements, surprisingly, use as much energy as surfing. It's all about posture, measured movement and control, and through its practice physical strength and health can be improved, along with balance and coordination. It provides a great, all-round physical and mental work out.

SWIMMING

Swimming is a lovely, low-impact exercise and is particularly good for protecting your joints, strengthening your muscles, improving your breath control and increasing stamina. It's also a total body and good cardiovascular exercise, which you can balance against other, higher-intensity exercises. Swimming is also a recognised stress buster, helping with focus and concentration. Its role in supporting breathing makes it a good exercise for those with asthma, too.

All you need is a swimming pool or access to the sea, a (safe) lake or river. Wild swimming is becoming increasingly popular, but requires some stoicism due to its colder temperatures – you may prefer a heated pool! Always make sure you swim somewhere safe, never alone or without the possibility of backup.

Although swimming is something anyone can learn or enjoy, if you are a poor or unconfident swimmer, a few classes will really help you get maximum benefit. Often, local pools run classes, or will have details of swimming coaches who can give you a few lessons.

WALKING

We are built for movement and the simplest exercise of all is walking – don't underestimate it! Factor in a little more walking every day, by opting to walk rather than taking the car, bus, train, tube or metro – even if that means getting off a stop or two before your destination. Even an extra 15 minutes a day will help – over the course of a working week, or the school run, that's over 2 hours of exercise you wouldn't otherwise have done; over 4 hours if you do it twice a day. And the health benefits will really start to pay off.

Walking is a weight-bearing exercise, so it has the added advantage of automatically maintaining or increasing bone density. Keeping our bones strong is particularly important as we age. It also helps maintain a healthy weight, but you need to walk briskly to ensure maximum benefit. This means walking at an energetic pace, where you are breathing hard but not gasping – you should just about be able to continue an intermittent conversation, but would probably find singing difficult!

You can improve the benefits of walking by swinging your arms as you walk, with or without small, hand-held weights. Nordic Walking – originally a summer training regime for cross-country skiers – is becoming increasingly popular as a form of total body exercise, with organisations, groups and instructors increasingly available to support you. Walking can be a very sociable activity, with walking workouts, walking groups, such as The Ramblers in the UK, or walking holidays and retreats available to try out. But the priority is just to walk, regularly, in a way that fits easily into your lifestyle.

RUNNING

Rather more than just brisk walking, running requires a bit of thought and proper footwear, although in theory you can do it anywhere. If you've never run before, you do need to take it gently at first, and build up stamina for distance and speed. It's high impact, hence the need for proper running shoes that will support the feet and protect the knees, as it can, over time, take its toll on both knees and hips.

Always do a few stretching exercises before you start, to warm up your muscles and reduce the risk of injury. As a novice runner, start by alternating walking and running. In the first week, begin with a brisk 5-minute warm-up walk, then alternate 1 minute of running with 2 minutes of walking, for a total of 20 minutes. Build incrementally from there. It's better to run little and often, rather than occasionally and for longer. By the end of 3 months, you should be able to run comfortably for 30 minutes, after a 5-minute warm-up.

Again, you can join running clubs to encourage and support you. You could train for a marathon, or just go for a gentle jog a couple of times a week to release stress, maintain a stable body weight and lift your mood.

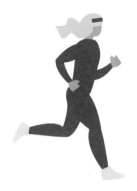

SPECIALIST
HELP

There's always a balance to be struck between exercise and the passivity that allows your body to rest and recuperate. You need to take enough exercise to keep everything working well and to avoid the injuries caused by a flabby musculature, repetitive strain or that ill-advised attempt to exceed your physical capabilities. A muscle that goes into spasm can be extremely painful and debilitating and demands your attention. Sometimes, an ice pack, some pain relief and rest will be enough, but other times you will need professional back-up, and an expert that specialises in the mechanics of the body will be your friend.

One of the benefits of external, hands-on treatments is that they can often help locate and identify problems, and then provide both treatment and self-help suggestions that can be very effective. Often, the emphasis is as much on what you can do to help yourself in general, following treatment of a specific complaint. The self-help recommendations will undoubtedly include exercise, to help strengthen muscles, which helps support the joints, tendons and ligaments.

PHYSIOTHERAPY

Trained in the function, mechanics and workings of the body, and its bones, muscles, tendons, ligaments and blood supply, physiotherapists have usually undergone a 3-year, degree-level training. They not only treat conditions such as sports injuries, sprains and strains, but also work to rehabilitate movement, mobility and function following injury or surgery. Many have additional training in massage or acupuncture, or other body therapies, to provide holistic treatment. They can also advise and recommend on exercise that you can – and must! – do, in order to aid your own recovery, and which will continue to support your health and fitness.

Following injury or surgery, your doctor may refer you to, or advise you see, a physiotherapist, but there is nothing to stop you self-referring, if you think this might be helpful. Their advice, for example, about gait, posture or exercise that will support your health, can be invaluable.

OSTEOPATHY

Many people see an osteopath regularly, for treatment or to maintain their physical health. It is a manual form of treatment designed to detect, treat and prevent musculoskeletal health problems. Often an osteopath's help is sought by those who have a bad back, but their expertise goes much further than that and treatment isn't limited to the high-velocity thrusts that are understood to be the tools of their trade. They also use very gentle manipulation, pressure and massage to ease pain and facilitate function. A fully trained osteopath, licensed to practise by an accredited body, is an expert in helping to restore and maintain function. Some may also have undertaken an additional 2-year training in paediatrics, enabling them to work safely on the youngest of infants, or may also have training in cranio-sacral work.

In the UK, osteopathy is considered an 'alternative' or 'complementary' treatment and only those registered with the General Osteopathic Council are allowed to call themselves osteopaths and practise clinically as such. In the USA, the profession is considered to be a branch of the medical profession and accredited as such. In Australia, osteopaths must be accredited to the Australasian Osteopathic Accreditation Council. So, wherever you are, check that your osteopath is properly qualified and accredited.

CHIROPRACTIC

This is another manual treatment of the musculoskeletal system, similar to osteopathy, but with more of a focus on treatment of the spine. It can be effective for some people with neck and lower back problems. Again, check your chiropractioner is properly trained, qualified and accredited with an official body.

MASSAGE

This can vary from light, rather superficial beauty massages, with lots of lovely aromatherapy oils, to rather more therapeutic sports massages. In the hands of a well-trained massage therapist, with a good knowledge of anatomy and physiology, a sports massage can be a very good way of releasing tension in the muscles and helping to relieve muscle spasm and reduce pain. It is particularly useful for deep muscles, such as the piriformis in the buttock, or in shoulder muscles that could impact on the neck. Physiotherapists and other professionals often have additional training in massage, which they can combine with their practice, and, if this is the case, they will probably be your best bet for a therapeutic massage. Sometimes, just releasing a muscle spasm with massage can be enough to reduce pain, and allow you the movement that will help you to stretch and strengthen your body to avoid further problems. Massage also restores blood flow to tired muscles, and can alleviate stiffness, through its external manipulation. Some massage therapists also extend their practice to include acupressure, shiatsu, or trigger-point therapy, where pressure is applied to specific areas of the body, which also help release muscle tension and spasm, and reduce energy congestion.

A study on the benefits of massage on chronic low back pain, carried out by the Group Health Research Institute and University of Washington, Seattle, in 2011, showed positive results, with its benefits '... about as strong as those reported for other effective treatments: medications, acupuncture, exercise and yoga,' according to Dan Cherkin, PhD, lead author of the study.

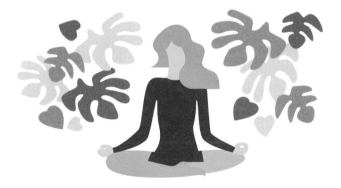

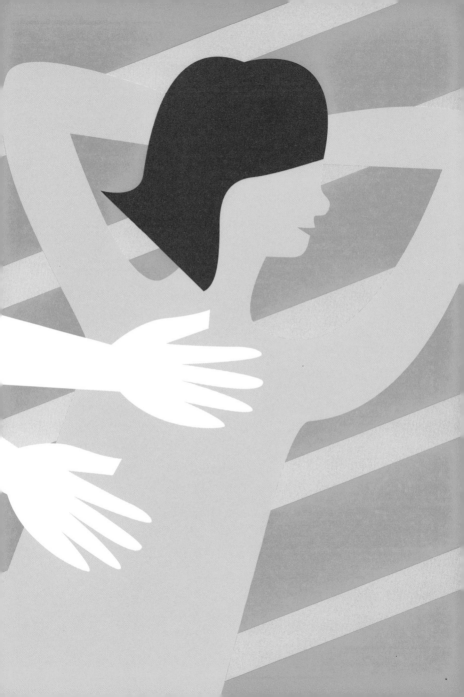

CONCLUSION

For anyone concerned about the physical problems that can arise from a sedentary lifestyle, the good news is that a lot can be done to counteract it and most of it is pretty simple: move frequently, stretch often and strengthen muscle tone.

MAKING TIME

Our busy lifestyles can mean we neglect our own health, so it's important to prioritise short, frequent breaks to counteract the impact of long hours spent sitting, and make these a routine feature. So, for example, get into the habit of rotating your neck and shoulders, and stretching your arms, while waiting for the kettle to boil; or discreetly clenching and unclenching your calf, thigh and buttock muscles, while waiting for a bus. When you walk anywhere, put your phone away, check your posture and walk briskly, gently swinging your arms. Use whatever time you have away from your chair to reconnect to your body. Use it, too, to reconnect to your breathing, connecting body and mind, heart and soul. Make it a habit and it will soon become a good one, and one that's hard to break.

HABIT FORMING

The jury's out on how long it takes to form a new habit. Back in the 1960s it was thought to be 21 days, but that's since been revised. It seems to vary from individual to individual, but, generally, you need to give it at least a month for a new habit to become familiar enough to stick with. It comes down to a variety of factors: your motivation, the ease with which you become familiar with what you need to do, etc. So give yourself the best chance by focusing on becoming familiar with the exercises, devising your own sequences that work for you, and feeling the benefit, for a good few weeks. Make exercising a priority until it just becomes as much a part of your day as cleaning your teeth.

Start Today and Feel Better Immediately

It's almost as simple as that!
And now you have the tools to do so,
you can do it.

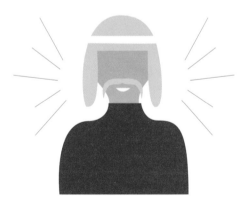

ACKNOWLEDGEMENTS

Many thanks, as ever, to the editorial team at Hardie Grant, in particular Kate Pollard, Kajal Mistry and Molly Ahuja for their diligence, patience and good humour through the writing of this book. Particular thanks are also due to designer and illustrator Evi Oetomo for doing such a great job.

It's a subject I feel very strongly about – as my two children will tell you – and because, as a writer, my life is very sedentary and I know how important it is to try and counteract its negative effects. In support of that, I have had huge hands-on benefit over the years from a wonderful physiotherapist Clare Whitaker, yoga teacher Carrie Rodd and osteopath Hedvig Verdonk, so a huge thank you to them, too. My posture isn't always the best, maybe, but it's way better than it might otherwise be!

ABOUT THE AUTHOR

Harriet Griffey is a journalist, writer and author of over 20 books, mostly focusing on health and wellbeing. She originally trained and worked as a state registered nurse, before moving into publishing and writing, and is the author of the highly acclaimed I Want to... series of books, also published by Hardie Grant.

I Want to Sleep

I Want to Be Calm

I Want to Be Organised

I Want to Be Happy

I Want to Be Confident

I Want to Be Creative

INDEX

Page numbers in *italics* refer to illustrations

Published in 2018 by Hardie Grant Books,
an imprint of Hardie Grant Publishing

Hardie Grant Books (London)
5th & 6th Floors
52–54 Southwark Street
London SE1 1UN

Hardie Grant Books (Melbourne)
Building 1, 658 Church Street
Richmond, Victoria 3121

hardiegrantbooks.com

British Library Cataloguing-in-Publication Data.
A catalogue record for this book is available
from the British Library.

Sit Strong by Harriet Griffey
ISBN: 978-1-78488-144-3

Publisher: Kate Pollard
Commissioning Editor: Kajal Mistry
Desk Editor: Molly Ahuja
Publishing Assistant: Eila Purvis
Art Direction: Evi O. / OetomoNew
Copy Editor: Emily Preece Morrison
Proofreader: Kay Delves
Colour Reproduction: p2d

*Every effort has been made to ensure that the content of
this book is accurate and safe but it is provided for general
information purposes only. If you have any concerns about your
health before starting any fitness programme, always consult
your doctor or medical practitioner.*

Printed and bound in China by 1010

Get your gears ready

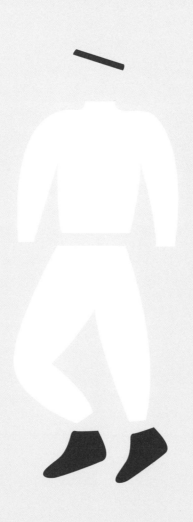

For my sons
Josh & Robbie